CRYSTAL BOBA

Discovering the Secret Ingredients to Making Fantastic Boba Drinks

Karen Robin

Contents

Introduction

Crystal boba, often referred to as "popping boba," is a well-liked and fashionable topping for frozen yogurt, bubble tea, and other sweets. It is manufactured from a combination of fruit juice, seaweed extract, and sodium alginate, as opposed to traditional boba, which is made from tapioca starch. This results in a thin outer layer that encases a burst of fruity liquid inside.

Although the outside of the crystal boba is chewy and soft and the juice within delivers a flavorful burst with each bite, the texture is distinctive and pleasurable to consume. Crystal boba is a flexible and eye-catching addition to any cuisine because it comes in a wide range of tastes like strawberry, mango, lychee, blueberry, and many more. Its versatility and color make it a vibrant accent to any recipe.

In addition to being enjoyable to consume, crystal boba is healthier than traditional boba since it contains fewer calories and less sugar. Crystal boba is also gluten-free and vegan, making it acceptable for anyone with dietary requirements.

Overall, the world of bubble tea and desserts has gained a tasty and inventive newcomer in the form of crystal boba. It is a well-liked option for people looking for a fresh take on their favorite snacks due to its distinctive texture and fruity flavors.

Chapter One

What is Crystal Boba?

Crystal Boba is another type of boba pearl used to brew boba tea. It is also referred to as "Agar Boba-flavored Taro Crystal Boba tea." These pearls are similar to other boba tea pearls yet stand out nonetheless. To be more precise, white agar powder-based boba pearls are what makeup crystal boba tea. Unknown to some, white agar is a gelling agent. This type of boba tea has a white tint because of the properties of white agar powder. Because of this and its modest transparency, it is known as "crystal boba." Crystal boba has a gelatinous texture like other varieties of boba tea.

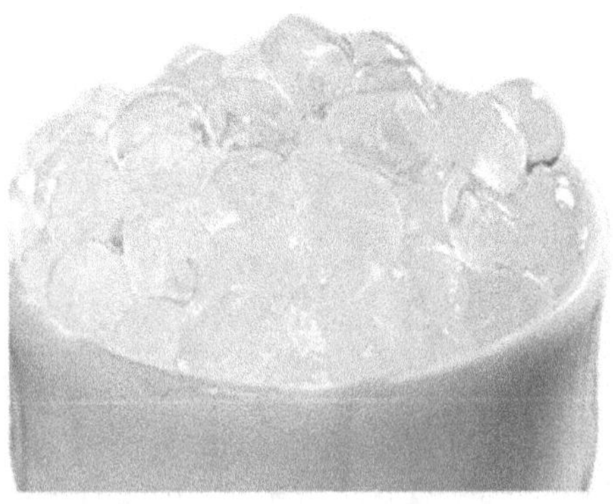

To offer crystal boba tea in a variety of flavors, it is typically pre-sweetened. This flavor can change to give you more options for drinks. The crystal pearls allow us to customize the hue of the boba. The tiny boba pearls at the bottom of boba tea are what give it its distinctive flavor. If these pearls weren't present, Boba tea would taste like any other iced tea or beverage. The boba tea pearls, which are bursting with flavor and give the beverage a distinctive consistency, give the drinker a break from monotonous textures. There are hundreds of distinct flavors and more than six different types of boba tea. The most well-liked boba tea varieties include milk tea, black tea, fresh milk, fruit tea and smoothies

Chapter Two

History of bubble tea

By adding tapioca pearls to her iced tea in 1988, Lin Hsiu Hui created the first pearl milk tea in Taiwan. Eventually, throughout the 1990s, Taiwanese immigrants brought it to the US.

At first, the only places to find bubble tea were Asian-American eateries. Bubble tea gained popularity in Los Angeles after Taiwanese immigrants started selling it there.

The East Coasters named the pearl milk tea "bubble tea," while those on the West Coast termed it "boba tea. "The terms "bubble" and "boba" both refer to the bubbles that appear on top of the beverage after shaking. Gelatinous chewy balls and milk- or fruit-based tea are combined to create bubble tea.

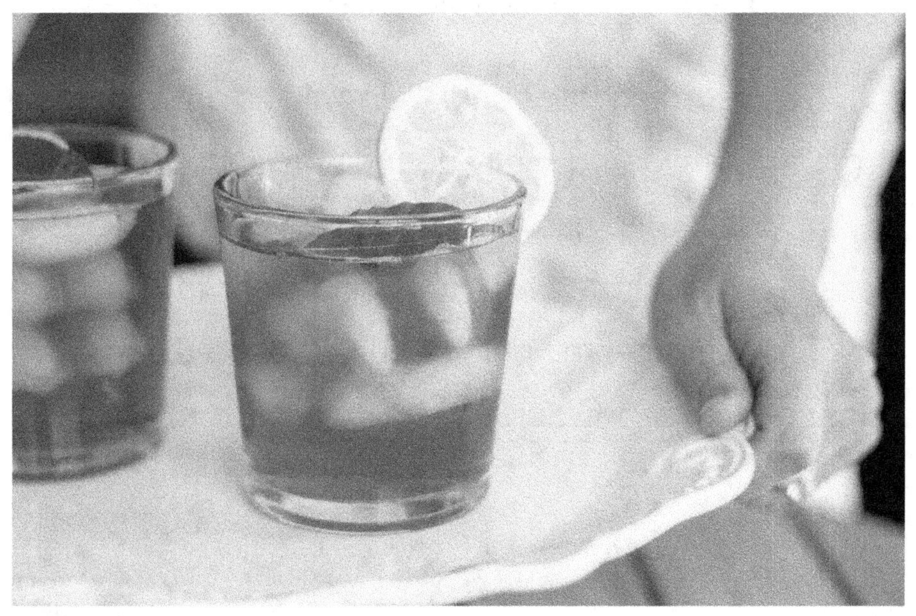

The image above shows the first pearl milk tea that was served by adding boba pearls on the iced tea.

Chapter Three

What are the components of crystal boba?

According to legend, the konjac plant, a tropical plant fsrequently found throughout Eastern Asia, is used to make crystal boba. But, because this plant is hard to find, individuals have developed simple recipes for crystal boba using white sugar and agar powder.

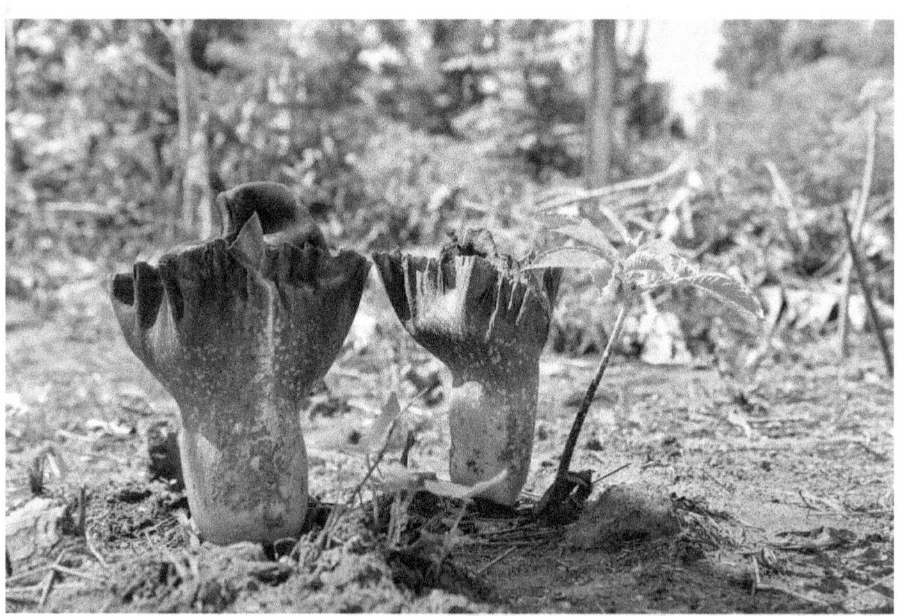

Chapter Four

What Flavor Does Crystal Boba Tea Have?

We simply mean crystal boba when we say crystal boba doesn't have much flavor. If all you ate were the chewy, gelatin-like crystal boba pearls. White pearls and agar boba are two names for crystal boba.

But because of their neutral flavor, we can use them to access the most incredible boba tea flavors. Crystal boba tea pearls can be used to make a creamy, fruity, sweet, and bright dish. Crystal boba pearls can be dipped in syrups with a pronounced sweetness to them. Sweet citrus fruit flavors are among the most widely used flavors. Grapefruit is a good illustration. The flavor of crystal boba is creamier when combined with milk. When combined with tea, though, it may taste more earthy. Almost anything goes, and soaking crystal boba in brown sugar is a popular trend.

Chapter Five
Regular Boba versus Crystal Boba

What sets crystal boba different from regular boba? In Asia, many concoctions incorporate both tapioca and white pearls. In contrast, the West mostly uses them for tea-based beverages. As a result, the differences between these two forms of boba are very well known, and each has a particular purpose. The typical bubble tea garnish used in the US and the UK is made of tapioca starch. The konjac plant is used to produce white pearls instead. The texture and taste of tapioca pearls are chewy and spongy. Compared to those used in other recipes, the tapioca pearls used in boba cocktails are frequently smaller and softer. Crystal boba, on the other hand, is incredibly soft and jelly-like. Because of the plant that is used to produce them, they also have a slight citrus flavor. After being put away or mixed into a beverage, white pearls retain their flavor as well.

On the other hand, tapioca pearls harden and begin to flavor the food around them. This could be advantageous or detrimental, depending on what you, the cook, intended to occur. Regular boba has a rich, opaque black color as a result of the caramel that is added during cooking. White pearls are distinctive and easy to identify since they are unmistakably white.

They are less common because of how noticeable they are. When added to a dish, crystal boba often becomes the main attraction. As a result, it is only used in teas and a few other limited treats.

Regular boba and crystal boba are both derived from the konjac plant, but normal boba is made from the starch of the tapioca root. Moreover, crystal boba has a transparent color, whereas conventional boba has a unique black hue. They both have modest flavors and chewy textures aside from that. The texture, flavor, nutrients, and preparation techniques of regular and crystal boba are distinct from one another. The ability to alter the hue of crystal boba is one of its distinctive features.

Regular boba can be made at home using tapioca starch and a variety of ingredients, just like crystal boba. Black and golden pearls are two of the most well-known regular boba varieties that people manufacture at home.

Chapter six

Crystal Boba versus Black Boba

Black Boba is a tapioca pearl that has been dyed a deep brownish-black by adding caramel or brown sugar. It is significantly sweeter than other forms of boba and has a licorice flavor. In the meantime, white sugar, agar powder, and coconut water are frequently used to make crystal boba. Although it isn't colored, people can add any food coloring they like to it to make it more interesting.

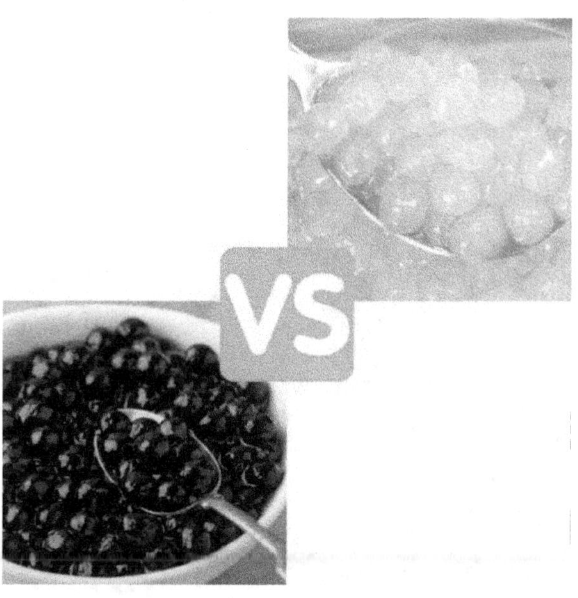

Chapter seven
Golden Boba versus Crystal Boba

Another version of tapioca pearls is known as "golden boba," but this time honey or golden food coloring has been added. It appeals to those with a sweet tooth because of its chewy texture and sweet flavor. The primary distinction between crystal boba and golden boba, besides color and flavor, is that the former has a more gelatinous texture due to the use of agar powder.

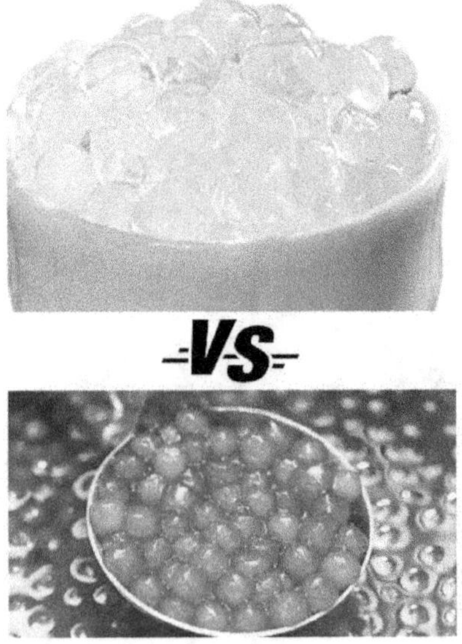

Chapter eight

Homemade Crystal Boba Recipe

Making crystal boba at home only requires a few simple components. You may expect a zesty touch to your tea because our recipe closely resembles the flavor of the original crystal boba. But first, let's talk about the ingredients before we get to the cooking. You need the following materials to produce crystal boba:

Coconut water, granulated sugar, vegetable oil, ice, agar powder, jelly powder, and squeeze bottles

Coconut Water:

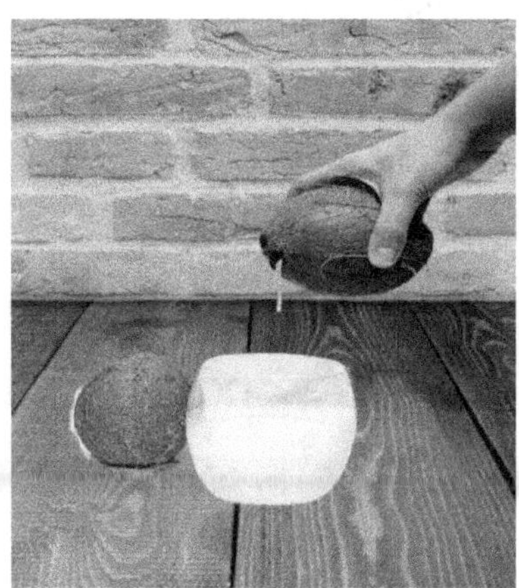

Konjac gum, which is hard to find outside of Eastern Asia, is primarily replaced by coconut water. It is an essential ingredient in every recipe for crystal boba because of its mild, tart flavor that resembles the Asian plant.

Agar Powder:

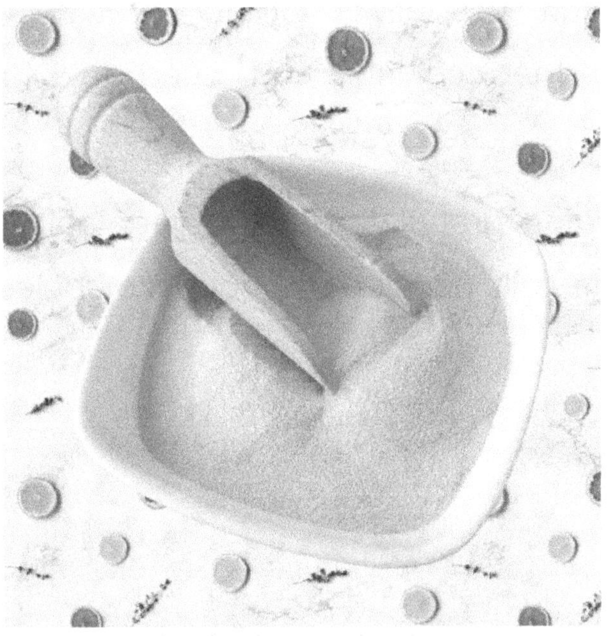

Agar is a jelly-like material that many recipes employ to stabilize and gelatinize foods. Crystal boba powder gives it a pleasantly gelatinous texture that is neither too jiggly nor too firm. It has no flavor or scent at all, making it the ideal addition to the recipe because it has no impact on the taste.

Jelly Powder:

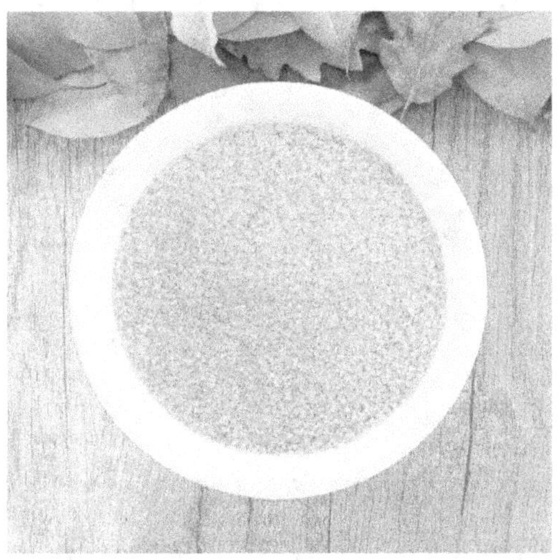

The crystal bubbles are gelatinized by agar powder, yet they do not acquire the chewy texture that boba tea drinkers often desire. The jelly powder is crucial in this situation since it gives the bubbles just the proper amount of chew. You can use any jelly flavor you like, but keep in mind that it needs to go well with the coconut water's citrus flavor.

Granulated Sugar:

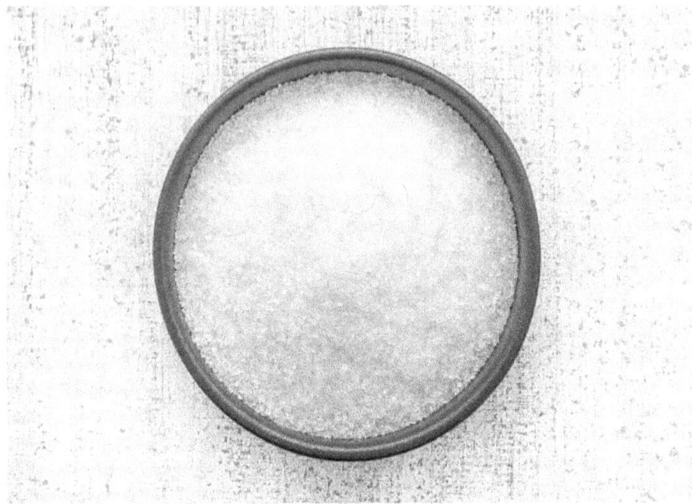

Now that there are components for crystal bubbles' flavor and texture, you still need one more for their distinctive crystal hue. It is best to use white powdered sugar because of its sweet flavor, which brings out the citrusy flavor of the bubbles and gives them a clear, white hue.

Vegetable Glycerin:

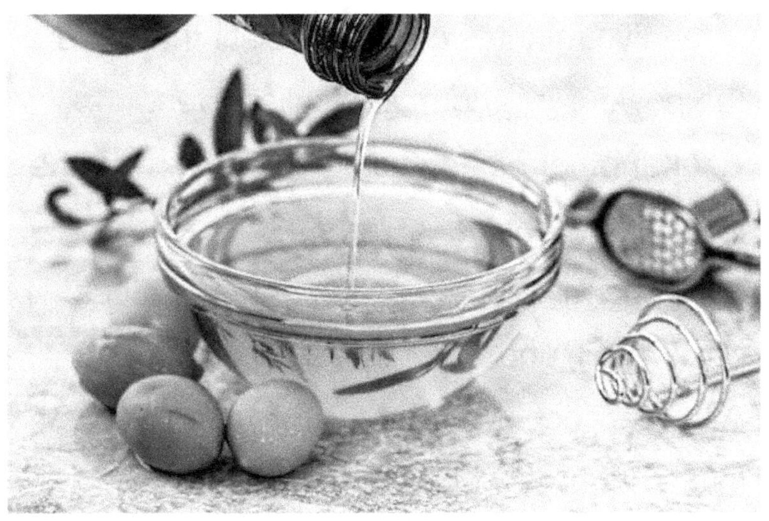

Vegetable oil is necessary to prevent the dish from clumping because vegetable boba has a lot of ingredients that can cling together while cooking.

Here is how to prepare home made recipe using the items we listed earlier in this chapter

1. Place a saucepan with the coconut water on low heat on the gas.
2. Next, combine the jelly and agar powder, add the mixture to the coconut water.

3. After five minutes of low heat, stir the mixture until the powder has completely dissolved.
4. After another 5 minutes of stirring, turn off the heat and remove the saucepan.
5. allow the mixture to cool for some minutes.
6. Mix ice, oil, and water in a sizable bowl.
7. After the coconut water mixture has cooled, pour it into a squeeze bottle.
8. Drop by drop, and squeeze the mixture into the sizable basin you previously prepared.
9. Watch the crystal bubbles until they reach the bowl's base. The bubbles should be strained and quickly rinsed.

After that, pour the mixture into a squeeze bottle and squeeze a little of it into the water mixture. The moment the pearls begin to drop to the bottom, you'll know they're ready.

After that, wash and filter them. The pearls that were removed are put in ice, or you can freeze them and keep them frozen for days. As a result, you can experiment with various tea flavors to see which ones best fit your palate. Typically, bubble milk boba is considered to go well with jasmine, lychee, and matcha. Original crystal pearls complement flavored iced teas well and add a wonderful texture to counteract the sweetness of the drink.

Chapter Nine

Benefits of Taking Crystal Boba

Consuming crystal boba is far healthier than other boba flavors. The majority of boba types are fat-free. They compensate for the absence of fat, which is excellent, with a greater calorie composition. Both are absent from crystal boba tea. Instead, this variety of boba has fewer calories and fats. The following are some possible advantages of consuming crystal boba:

Fewer Calories:

Compared to regular boba, which is produced from tapioca starch, crystal boba typically has fewer calories. This makes it a fantastic choice for folks who are calorie conscious. Crystal boba has fewer calories than other bubble tea toppings like tapioca pearls. A healthier alternative for individuals watching their calorie intake, crystal boba typically has 10 to 15 calories per spoonful.

Rich in Fiber:

The fiber-rich seaweed extract used to manufacture crystal boba can aid in the promotion of digestive health and the prevention of constipation.

High in Vitamins and Minerals:

Fruit juice, which is frequently used to make crystal boba and is an excellent source of vitamins and minerals like vitamin C, potassium, and folate.

Has Antioxidants:

A number of the fruits used to make crystal boba are high in antioxidants, which can enable the body to battle off free radicals and reduce the likelihood of chronic illnesses. For instance, blueberry-based boba contains a lot of antioxidants that can help shield your body from the harm that free radicals can do.

Adds a Flavorful Burst:

Crystal boba is a popular addition to drinks because of its excellent flavor and distinctive texture. They come in many flavors, including lychee, mango, strawberry, and others, and when you bite into them, they give off a chewy, juicy burst.

Chapter ten

Where Can You Buy Crystal Boba?

Crystal boba is relatively simple to obtain. This kind of boba tea is often available at most grocery stores and boba businesses. You'll probably find it at most pop-up boba cafes as well. You could even use crystal boba to produce your boba tea if you're prepared to put in the work. There are so many sources of crystal boba that you can even purchase the pearls in grocery shops and online. We suggest going on Amazon if you want to buy some crystal boba pearls online. There are a lot of reliable sellers of ready-to-wear crystal boba pearls on Amazon. After you have the pearls, making your own crystal boba tea just requires a small number of additional ingredients.

Final Reflections

We've discussed what crystal boba is and how it tastes in this book. As we've already demonstrated, crystal boba doesn't truly have much flavor on its own. We also discussed how the basic flavor of this particular variety of boba makes it one of the most adaptable. We also included how to make your own boba pearls. Now that you are fully informed about crystal boba, why not try producing some yourself or purchasing some to see how it looks like? Try out several flavors to find which ones you prefer.